Why Not? Thoughts About Crossdressing and Male Feminization

by Barbara Deloto and Thomas Newgen

TABLE OF CONTENTS

Why Not?

Many times something fun isn't always *good* for you. Well, hobbies can be beneficial for everyone, relieving stress, widening our interests, satisfying basic human needs, and helping us grow as people. Abraham Harold Maslow established a hierarchy of human needs, and hobbies in general and this particular hobby, of cross-dressing, is very good at satisfying them, as we'll see later.

Google the word "cross-dressing" and you'll find there are 16,200,000 hits. It's huge! Google "dresses for men" and there are 74,800,000 hits! "Men's dresses and skirts" yields 17,300,000 results. It may be something that isn't often talked about or shared openly, but it's a huge market for products and a huge, worldwide community.

We all have traits and aspects of both genders within us. There are no purely masculine or purely feminine persons. One may think they are one or the other, but the reality is different, and it's essential for to it be that way. What would a dad be without the feminine nurturing trait? How can a woman be successful if she doesn't utilize her power as an individual and is instead always submissive. The idea of pure gender is a cultural construct, and if it were to exist, the world would be all messed up.

The Kybalion was first published in 1908 by the Yogi Publication Society and is now in the public domain. Based on ancient Hermeticism, the publication early on makes the claim that *The Kybalion* makes its appearance in one's life when the time is appropriate—very much like the saying that goes, "When the student is ready, the teacher appears." The book reveals seven basic laws that form a philosophy of life, which has been utilized as guiding principles since it's publication, and is still very prevalent today. A proper understanding and application of these laws, according to the text, will allow an individual to achieve self-mastery.

One of the seven laws in *The Kybalion* is the law of gender. The concept states that gender exists on all planes of existence (physical, mental, and spiritual). Everything and everyone contain both masculine and feminine elements or principles. The feminine principle is always in the direction of receiving impressions and has a more varied field of operation than the masculine. The feminine generates new thoughts, concepts, and ideas, including the work of the imagination.

The masculine principle is always in the direction of giving out or expressing; it concerns itself with the "will" in its varied phases.

The book says there must be a balance between these two forces. Without the feminine, the masculine is apt to act without restraint, order, or reason, resulting in chaos. The feminine alone, in contrast, is apt to constantly reflect and fail to act, resulting in stagnation. When the masculine and feminine work together, however, thoughtful action creates success, because the feminine and the masculine fulfill each other.

Masculine and feminine both live within each of us. Women taking on masculine aspects can rise to powerful leadership positions and overcome repression and submission. Today they can carry male power within them without any problem in society. Men are not always as fortunate when their feminine aspects are revealed.

However, when a male becomes feminized, it can open doors to a greater understanding and utilization of a male's inherent, though sometimes repressed, feminine nature. A new worldview can be gained, allowing reflection and consideration of a newfound wholeness of being. So, why not?

First, let's look at some thoughts about this particular hobby, cross-dressing and feminization. Are you bored male or do you know one who's looking for something new to do? Someone who's tired of the same old stuff? Well, here's a hobby a guy can really engage in. It's only for the courageous man, a real man who isn't afraid of trying new thing—a man that can let go of his masculinity for a time and not let it damage his ego. Excess spare time, boredom and stress, will be taken care of if he can find it in himself to indulge in this new exploration and growth.

We've previously written a how-to book on the feminizing process to give interested men, or people wishing to feminize their man, a strong start on this road of exploration, and make them their feminine best as soon as possible. Now we write on the benefits for those males who may be on the edge of discovery but yet to do it, or those males fully engaged in the practice already, or those women interested in something new to explore for the male *they* know.

Taking a walk on the wild side, so to speak, has never been easier or more fun. With the advent of online shopping, millions of males have begun actively and passionately engaging in this hobby, which takes away their troubles and gives them something to look forward to when they aren't at work. Large communities have sprung up on the internet, connecting like-minded people, and the cross-dressing community is no different. Not everyone who indulges in this pastime will join a club, but just Google "cross-dressing clubs" and you'll see there are 885,000 hits, with clubs everywhere. Although it's secretive for most who do it, it certainly isn't an obscure hobby.

"But I'm a married guy," you say. "What will my wife think?" Well of course, if you're married, you have to consider your spouse. She may be looking at it as something freakish and unmanly rather than considering the benefits for both of you. You'll have to discuss it with her if you want her to share in the activity, or not discuss it with her and keep it your own private secret as many men do. Either way, it can still be a source of great pleasure, entertainment, and even growth.

She may say, "A *real* man would never try to look like a woman." Many *real* men in the armed services, heads of companies, responsible and intelligent men all over the world, indulge in the pleasure of turning themselves into something sensual and pretty that gives them a new view of the world. It takes courage for them to face the fact that we are all made up of male and female aspects, and explore their feminine side. Many men would never risk damaging their male ego to try it. The courageous ones have put aside paradigms and beliefs, along with their male egos, and stepped into the icy water of change to become something special beyond their wildest dreams. It takes a *real* man to be able to do it.

"Why would a real man want to waste time trying to act and look like a woman. Why would a guy ever want to do such a thing?" you say.

The experience. Cross-dressing males, once they've done it, usually continue for a number of reasons. The biggest reason is how good it makes them feel, and it can be a fantastic diversion from the mundane world. It relieves stress better than most anything, and does so without drugs, alcohol, nicotine, or pills of any kind. It harms no one and provides something to plan for and look forward to.

And you say very pragmatically, "Women's clothes and shoes are expensive, and women always buy so much. It isn't prudent."

It doesn't cost much compared to other pastimes and hobbies. The clothes can be bought on EBay or other inexpensive clothing sites as well as in local thrift shops. High heels as well. Of course one can shop in pricier venues, but it isn't necessary. Compare that to flying drones, hunting trips, photography equipment, biking gear, golf equipment and fees, skiing and so on, which can run up the bills tremendously and aren't always as convenient, safe, or easy to do.

"Guys are too big to look like women." Maybe some are. But that won't keep the guy from feeling like a totally new person. There are large women, too, and some large men look better dressed *en femme* than some large women do, because they pay attention to details a normal woman wouldn't bother with. Once a man learns what works for him, he'll have a whole new persona to indulge in anytime.

If a guy is one of the lucky, shorter males, though, he'll likely be able to feminize *so well* that it's highly plausible he could go out in public, and no one would even know. Imagine the thrill of a feminized male going out in public, presenting as a woman who is going shopping for a new dress or other item. Talk about a leap of courage!

Imagine the feeling of accomplishment being able to dress and act like the graceful, elegant, or even sexy opposite gender, and to be treated like one… Doors opening for her, compliments, winks, smiles, all the while immersed in the indulgence of femininity, while shopping, eating out, clubbing, or just going for a walk.

Will that happen for you or your hobbyist? Maybe, maybe not. Even if one who forgoes going in public and does nothing more than lounge at home in sensual splendor, being something totally different, and escaping the mundane, stress-filled world for a while, wouldn't that be worth it? Many men have come to the conclusion that it absolutely is.

If you're in a male-female relationship and you're both open-minded people, cross-dressing can enhance it. You'll have many things to share—tastes in clothing, shopping, cuddling together, being best friends, and maybe even a more exciting sex life. Once the doorway has been opened, paradigms are broken, and it's accepted as a way to enhance a relationship and bring joy to you both, it can be a marvelous time for each of you.

The barriers of gender roles disappear. How nice to have you both sharing in household tasks, cooking, shopping, and so on! You do all things together, sharing time pursuing a mutual interest. He may even take on what were previously her duties in order to please her, making the experience better for both.

How nice to have a totally hygienic male that always smells nice with no body hair to accumulate sweat and stink, and is neat and clean, whether feminine or masculine that day! No more mono-brow or bushy, unkempt eyebrows. Clean and neat fingernails and toenails. Attention given to skin and hair, and maybe even weight watching to be able to fit into her favorite skirt.

Perfume lingering in the closet from *en femme* times versus the stinking sweat from sporting pastimes or the reek of fishing gear. Many women love the changes they never would have predicted once the hobbyist learns to be their feminine best.

Why Not?

The changes won't be evident solely when *en femme*. They'll carry into masculine time as well. Even then you can both enjoy shopping together and pursuing your mutual new hobby together. She'll be motivated to help get things ready for the weekends so both of you can enjoy a fine meal and drinks together and maybe a night of cuddling and hot sex.

There will be a reason for you both to get a new dress or outfit to enjoy, rather than lying around in shorts and sweats and watching the game on TV. The hobbyist will view previous pastimes such as poker night with the guys as boring in comparison, allowing more time to share together. Rather than two roommates with separate pastimes, you'll be two BFFs with the same interests, both looking forward to the next time to share together. If there is no partner, the hobbyist can still indulge in it, having wonderful relaxing experiences.

So whether you're a woman in a relationship with man, a man in a relationship with a woman, or two males in a relationship together, or a sole practitioner, what harm can come from exploring a safe and delightful entertainment? It doesn't have to be made public (but it can be), and there's a whole community out there to join if desired—communities with sole practitioners and communities with couples.

So turn those male toenails into pretty women's toenails and dip those pretty feet into the icy cold water of excitement and exploration, then indulge in a pastime that will entertain, de-stress, and relax you for years to come. Why not?

Hmm. Maybe you're repulsed by all of this, and it just won't work for you or your significant other due to your paradigms and beliefs—your rigid view of how things are meant to be just won't allow it. Go ahead. Quit. Do nothing and stay on your treadmill where it's safe, and maybe boring, and maybe mundane, and commonplace—where time stands still while life and exploration slide by. Let others explore and brave the titillation of change and growth. Toss this book aside and don't give it a second thought.

Or turn the page and find out more about how a person can grow from it.

Maslow's Hierarchy

Abraham Harold Maslow (1908–1970) was an American psychologist best known for creating Maslow's hierarchy of needs, a theory of psychological health based on fulfilling innate human needs in priority, resulting in self-actualization. He was a psychology professor at Brandeis University, Brooklyn College, and Columbia University. He stressed the importance of focusing on people's positive qualities. A *Review of General Psychology* survey, published in 2002, ranked Maslow as the tenth most cited psychologist of the 20th century.

When one looks at his hierarchy of needs and sees where cross-dressing fits in, it becomes all the more obvious why so many men are doing it today. I'm certain they aren't motivated to do it in order to fulfill the hierarchy, but rather they do it *naturally*—and the hierarchy reflects *human nature*, because the hierarchy reflects *each and every person's* nature. It's *human nature* that drives one to fulfill Maslow's hierarchy of human needs, and male-to-female cross-dressing is a hobby that can nurture the individual's development in their search for Maslow's highest attainment on the hierarchy—self-actualization.

We often see cases in which a hobby carries over to the rest of life. Someone interested in technical things may build and fly drones, work on cars or other vehicles, build and create things in their spare time. When they do so, they may carry that learning and experience into their daily lives and further enhance their professional pursuits.

Others may be interested in team sports and apply the concept of teamwork to their daily work. Still others may be highly analytical, planning out sequences of events and may have chess as a hobby, which gives them patterns and a sense of sequencing to incorporate into their lives.

The hobby of cross-dressing may have as much, if not more, impact on personal achievement at the highest level of Maslow's hierarchy than many men's hobbies and interests. The men who engage in cross-dressing probably never even thought about it, because it was so natural to them to pursue it once they began.

Many men who cross-dress are intelligent and successful in life. Is that because they were successful to begin with, giving them the open and inquisitive mind to pursue it, or is their success in life a result coupled to their pursuit of cross-dressing. What came first, the chicken or the egg? It may be both.

It may have started as a fetish, or a simple interest in things feminine, or as a suggestion or mandate from a partner, but it ends up for many as a way to grow, feel, and express things they'd never imagined. It impacts their non-fem days and lives and develops them as a human being—growing and rising through Maslow's hierarchy of need fulfillment.

As we work our way through the different things that happen when men become feminized and present themselves as a female as a hobby, we'll refer to Maslow's levels as a reference to see where on the pyramid it's associated. Join us as we climb Maslow's pyramid of need fulfillment.

Basic Needs

The physiological needs are at the first level of the hierarchy. These are very basic needs; everyone has them, and they *must* be fulfilled before we can consider higher-level needs. Food, water warmth, and anything related to the health of the physical body aids in meeting physiological needs.

Safety and security are in the second level. Unfortunately, in today's world, a feminized male might reduce their safety and security by being caught in public by the more primitive and prejudiced beings in society. Society is what it is, though it isn't as bad as in the past. One day it may not be an issue at all. Our discussion here will concentrate on what can be capitalized on rather than what can't.

However, safety and security are feelings many cross-dressing males *obtain* when they are *en femme*. Cross-dressing is a haven of relaxation and escape for them. No callings from the male world make it through to their fem-selves. They leave all the threatening, stressful aspects of their male lives far behind to immerse themselves in a feeling of safety and security in their fem identities. Their fem self doesn't face responsibilities, answer her boss, or even work. She has nothing to fix or take care of, unlike her male side, except maybe a piece of her jewelry or a heel on her shoe. She's all about feeling good and being herself, not even thinking about her male half's problems. She is totally stress-free.

When a male takes an interest in cross-dressing and pursues it, it can bring incomprehensible pleasure. There's the dip into increased sensuality from things like having a silky, shaved body that feels the caress of sheer stockings, silky panties, and dresses, the tug of gel breast-forms on the chest. There's walking in the high heels, which shorten her stride, making her feel deliciously vulnerable and sexy and making her hips sway with each step, and the allure of her perfumed body and long, painted nails and toenails. It all immerses cross-dressers into sensations they would never experience presenting as a male, and opens them up to heretofore unrealized pleasures.

What happens when a person feels *that good* and *sensual*? Endorphins flood their brain. It's similar to the rush a marathon runner experiences, but without the stress and strain on the body. The endorphins reduce stress, ward off anxiety and feelings of depression, boost self-esteem, and improve sleep. The overall physiological self is nurtured and refreshed.

The immediate effect is a feeling of pleasure and a sense of deep satisfaction. All of these things are critical for humans if they are to have enjoyable lives, to be capable of driving forward to bigger and better things on their way up the pyramid of the hierarchy.

Can endorphins be created in other ways? Of course, but cross-dressing is much simpler, and the likelihood of any physical damage, especially compared to the strenuous physical activity that typically produces them, is much less. Not to mention, how sensual does running or heavy physical activity feel compared to the sensation of the feminized male's skin against the silky fabrics and the sensuality of their feminized walk and actions? Not only do they create plenty of feel-good endorphins easily, they also get to experience other pleasures that running or working out will never give, and without sore muscles.

The relaxed and de-stressed body of a cross-dresser can have reduced blood pressure thanks to their improved physiology. A calming peacefulness drops the heart rate and blood pressure to induce a feeling similar in effect to meditation or deep relaxation. Not a bad thing, either, in this high-stress world that just seems to boost our blood pressure.

What other physical improvements are there for a male-to-female cross-dresser? How about improved libido? Someone who is stressed and depressed is unlikely to be very interested in sex and could possibly have erectile dysfunction (ED).

From the Mayo Clinic, here are the psychological reasons for ED: "The brain plays a key role in triggering the series of physical events that cause an erection, starting with feelings of sexual excitement. A number of things can interfere with sexual feelings and cause or worsen erectile dysfunction. These include:

- Depression, anxiety or other mental health conditions
- Stress
- Relationship problems due to stress, poor communication, or other concerns

With the flow of endorphins and the pleasant state of mind cross-dressing creates, these things drift away, allowing the experience of heightened libido and sexual satisfaction—all without a pill!

Other physical benefits come from, as mentioned earlier, the higher level of hygiene required to transform from a male presentation to a female one. The body is shaved clean, and the skin is moisturized and silky. Dry patches disappear, and the skin is scrutinized regularly while shaving and caring for it. Body odor drops in the absence of body hair to collect sweat and odor, and the sweaty places for funguses to thrive are gone. The person has a renewed sense of what it's like to be clean and fresh and has a hobby that keeps them that way.

Walking in heels? Hmm, that has to be bad, right? Not necessarily. The shifted posture in heels can provide relief to the spine by allowing it to hold a new position from the one it would have in flat-heeled shoes. This can allow the spine to flex and move and strengthen the back muscles to provide greater support when not in heels.

Improving spinal alignment is what chiropractors do for a living, and high heels can possibly provide that as well. I've known men who have experienced relief from their sciatica when fully feminized. Whether it be from the endorphins, the stretching and bending while shaving their legs, or brief spinal relief from the high heels, it's something they enjoy as a benefit.

Another physical improvement that shows up consistently once men are regularly feminizing themselves is the desire to improve their appearance as a woman. Many of them improve their diets, eating better foods and watching their weight, reducing their chance of diabetes and other health issues, and improving their overall health and well-being.

As all women know, women hate it when they can't wear a favorite article of clothing, whether it be a skirt or dress, and this helps the cross-dresser to pay closer attention to their diet and weight. One instance of not being able to zip a favorite skirt, and the red flag pops up and drives a change.

In total, there is little or no risk of reducing physiological performance of a feminized male, and in most cases there is *improved* physiological performance from the endorphins and the inherent nature of the process of fully feminizing oneself to present as a woman. No sore muscles or pulled backs from working out. No damaged knees or feet from running. No funguses from locker rooms or accumulated sweat on the body. No hunting accidents.

Instead, there is an improved physiological state with a lasting hobby to keep it that way and a more hygienic presentation when not *en femme,* carrying with it an improved state of mind and health.

Once the physiological needs are met, a person *naturally* strives to achieve the next level of Maslow's hierarchy, the psychological needs. Wow. How can this be? This hobby sounds like a miracle pill. Well, it practically is. Now let's talk about psychological need fulfillment.

Psychological Needs Fulfillment

The third and fourth levels in Maslow's hierarchy are the psychological needs of the individual. Anything that can influence and improve the level of psychological fulfillment gives the person another step up the pyramid of needs. A feminized male can fulfill many psychological needs without the aid of drugs of any sort, exclusively by pursuing their hobby.

We already talked about stress and depression and their effects at the physiological level, but they carry over into the psychological level, manifesting in detrimental behaviors. But this isn't the only psychological advantage a feminized male gains from his hobby. Its positive influence is as widespread as women's clothing styles and options for his new look.

A male who feminizes himself regularly uses his time differently than before. When one has nothing interesting and exciting to do, they become bored. Boredom leads to a reduction in the physiological realm and the psychological realm as well. Overall health diminishes. Love for life is gone. Time seems to stand still.

Below is the summary from "Bored to death?" by Annie Britton and Martin J. Shipley of the Department of Epidemiology and Public Health, University College London, London, UK, published in the *International Journal of Epidemiology*, Volume 39, Issue 2, 1 April 2010, Pages 370–371, https://doi.org/10.1093/ije/dyp404:

> We conclude that those who report being bored are more likely to die younger than those who are not bored. However, the state of boredom is almost certainly a proxy for other risk factors. Whilst some aspects of life may not be so easily modified (e.g. disease status or position in society), proneness to boredom, particularly in younger populations, could

be indicative of harmful behaviours such as excessive drinking, smoking, taking drugs and low psychological profiles. Finding renewed interest in social and physical activities may alleviate boredom and improve health, thus reducing the risk of being 'bored to death.'

Regular feminization as a hobby becomes a passion that doesn't allow for boredom. There's no time to be bored when looking for the next outfit, that perfect top, or the earrings that will go with the new necklace. There's no time to be bored when the house needs to be readied for the glorious weekend of indulgence in endorphin-boosting. The extra time spent on hygiene and body care takes time that might otherwise be spent lying on the couch or looking for a diversion such as watching porn or sports.

Let's not forget to mention, if the hobbyist has a partner with whom to share this gift, they will both be able to share in the entertainment of maximizing the hobbyist's appearance and feminization. Neither of them can become bored when driven by this desire to excel.

When a person has a full life, their discretionary time filled with a joyful pastime, their mindset becomes one of optimism and willingness to overcome. The optimism gives them the strength to overcome other obstacles in their daily lives by knowing they will regularly have fulfillment and great pleasure. Every day, the trivial and mundane are taken care of and moved past quickly and efficiently in order to maximize the enhancement of this life and its rewards.

There aren't aching muscles saying you really don't want to run on the treadmill. There isn't frustration that the weather isn't allowing you to go hunting, fishing, or golfing. It can rain all it wants; it doesn't matter. The feminized male hobbyist knows they will be able to pursue their pleasure no matter what, and their optimism is all the more present in this knowledge.

There is *always* another fun and rewarding time to look forward to, even in the preparations and obtaining desired accoutrements, and these enjoyable tasks can be done whenever there's a small block of time available. When partners plan together for a special weekend or night together, the effect drifts from one of them to the other, with mutual benefits coming from the hobbyist's pursuits.

As time goes on, as in any other pursuit, practice makes perfect. Just the right hairstyle is found, just the right makeup, the perfect style and fit of clothing, the preferred heel height and favorite brand of stockings. The perfect perfume lifts the senses as it's spritzed over silky legs, under her skirt and in her hair, signaling the start of another fine evening.

Pictures may be taken for reflection and perfection. Time goes on, and the illusion becomes better and better. Self-esteem rises from the accomplishment and attainment, which in turn, like any other dedicated pursuit, builds confidence and the desire to continually improve.

Attainment and overcoming fears and reservations shrinks the amygdalae in the brain and gives control to the prefrontal cortex. The amygdalae grow with anger, fear, and stress when a person doesn't accomplish, and the reverse happens when they do accomplish. Inevitably, feminized males accomplish what they set out to do even if they aren't a perfect reflection of a feminine and petite woman. The satisfaction they gain gives them a feeling of accomplishment. The amygdalae shrink and the prefrontal cortex is more available for cognitive pursuits.

Below is from book, *The Marshmallow Test: Mastering Self-Control* by Walter Mischel. He is an Austrian-born American psychologist specializing in personality theory and social psychology and the Robert Johnston Niven Professor of Humane Letters in the Department of Psychology at Columbia University. A *Review of General Psychology* survey, published in 2002, ranked Mischel as the 25th most cited psychologist of the 20th century. From *The Marshmallow Test* comes this:

After reviewing research on the effects of stress, neuroscientist Amy Arnsten at Yale University concluded, "even quite mild acute uncontrollable stress can cause a rapid and dramatic loss of prefrontal cognitive abilities." The longer stress persists, the more those cognitive abilities are hurt and the more permanent the damage, ultimately leading to a mental as well as physical illness. Thus, the part of the brain that enables creative problem-solving becomes less available the more we need it.

The corollary is also true. The more the prefrontal cortex is used, the smaller the amygdalae's influence becomes, and their ability to rule a person is diminished. Fear of failure, unfounded fears, anger, and so on, diminish. Cross-dressing males relieve stress, attain goals, and engage in creativity, reducing the amygdalae and making the prefrontal cortex more powerful. The cross-dressing male again moves further up Maslow's pyramid because of his indulgence in this hobby.

For some cross-dressing males, the level of attainment of presenting as a woman brings great pride and longing to share this attainment with other like-minded people. They may join clubs or blogs, meet others like them, share techniques, products, and methods, and become part of a larger community where they are accepted and even admired by women who love them, and men who don't cross-dress themselves.

Online clubs such as URNOTALONE.com or Crossdresser Heaven.com give members a place to meet, communicate, share, and be a part of the community. They provide resources and articles and a place to belong. There are many more online and actual clubs for the cross-dresser interested in being a part of it. Find them all simply by Googling, joining Facebook clubs and so on.

There are conventions where hundreds of fully feminized males go singly or with their partners or spouses for a vacation to be with others like themselves or admirers. They attend workshops for learning, dinners and dances, public outings, and other events and contests. Some of these gatherings are week-long, others a weekend, but they take place in many locations that can be found simply by Googling *crossdresser conference.*

There are places to post fiction and read others' stories as well. There are blogs for discussion. Once one sees how much there is out there, it becomes obvious how popular it is.

Sometimes miles are crossed to meet each other, or the street is crossed when one finds out who else is partaking in this hobby through a local or worldwide club. The psychological needs of belonging and the needs for love as well as esteem and accomplishment bring the cross-dresser higher yet on the pyramid, to be near the apex of self-actualization, and self-fulfillment

They can reach a point of gratification and fullness in life that may have eluded them before. What is more creative than trying to pick out outfits as a woman? There is a plethora of colors, fabrics, and styles, all that have to be mated with the proper shoes, purses, hairstyle, jewelry, lipstick, eyeshadow, nail polish and so on. The number of variables that can be combined to create a theme or style for the feminized male for a single night can be shocking compared to what a their male self may decide upon to get dressed.

How much creativity do other hobbies allow? Running? Working out? Not even close. A whole new level of creativity is achieved, and that same creativity carries over in some shape and form into their daily lives as well.

Then, once they have delved so deeply into this new endeavor, they may even achieve transcendence, whereby they are motivated by values that rise above the personal self. For example, mystical experiences, experiences with nature, aesthetic experiences of course (feminization is all about aesthetics), sexual experiences (possibly a new view on gender and the investigation of the true nature of the sexual being versus society's rigid borders and barriers), service to others, and the pursuit of other new and now intriguing investigations and learning. The mind flies open as paradigms crash and the world's interconnectedness is revealed as the veil is lifted. (Or worn as a bride in a theme night's fantasy for her).

The act of engaging in this pursuit can be a form of spiritual zazen, a Zen Buddhist practice. All other thoughts and judgements fall away, leaving the participant immersed in the moment, allowing them to put aside other thoughts and concerns.

So, looking at Maslow's hierarchy, we see that there are a number of things that can be obtained from the diligent pursuit by a passionate hobbyist on the road to exploring a male's feminine side. It can be an avenue to achieve the highest levels of human attainment, rising and growing in Maslow's hierarchy of human needs and delivering to the hobbyist immense personal gratification with carryover into their regular male lives.

If your partner has in some way shown interest in such a pursuit, if you yourself have thought about it but not had the courage to do it, if you know someone who cross-dresses, or if you already do it, now you have some insight into what it can mean to a person beyond simply pleasure. You can see how much of a benefit it can be to them and to others as well.

Their courage in walking this taboo path, where the bulk of society derides the walker and belittles them, has the potential for turning them into much more than they may have been before, and they should be held in high esteem if not respected and loved.

Whether it is the cross-dressing that has done it, or the fact that the individual was already there before they began, the cross-dressing male tends to be more intelligent, caring, and open-minded than purely masculine males and they are usually quite successful in their regular daily lives—attributes we all should strive to achieve.

So, why not?

Ready to begin? You may ask, "What will it be like?"

What Will It Be Like?

Who are you? A spouse? A partner or girlfriend? A walker on the path of cross-dressing? No matter who you are, it's likely that initially there will be an internal struggle with our societal paradigms. *This isn't right. This is unnatural. This is deviant behavior.* But where do those feelings originate?

They originate where all prejudice, hate, derisive comments, and judgement of others originate. From fear. People's amygdalae see something as different or not understandable, and since they can't quickly identify with it, they see it as threatening. The amygdalae kick into gear and override the prefrontal cortex, the center of higher cognitive abilities, and tell the person with strong and loud shouts, "This is bad! They are bad! They are a threat!"

This is no different than any hate group, supremacist organization, or governing powers such as religions, the military, or a nondemocratic government trying to control a population. They fear that allowing one to delve into an area perceived to be different will create more deviance and will threaten society or the individual. All of their actions come not from the prefrontal cortex, but from their amygdalae, the reptilian brain meant to protect beings from danger. In their need to be a part of the greater whole or at least to be perceived as that (that is another of Maslow's hierarchy needs—acceptance) they follow the lemmings' decisions of right and wrong and their amygdalae.

So, the friend, spouse, partner or sole practitioner of this practice probably can and will hear those voices. Guilt, shame, fear, ego, masculine image, all are threatened by the simple act of being in touch with a male's feminine self. Whatever viewpoint it comes from, it will probably be there.

Not to worry. Unless the participant plans on living daily life this way, the fear is unfounded, and once put aside by using the prefrontal cortex for cognitive thinking, the truth can be seen. Some may choose to pursue a daily life *en femme,* and society is becoming more understanding, but the struggle remains due to all the reptilian portions of people's brains sparking them into action. As understanding grows, fear and the amygdalae's responses will leave the prefrontal cortexes to take charge and support rather than destroy.

In the much smaller realm of private lives, where the closest of friends and lovers are concerned, simply putting aside paradigms and beliefs and supporting the brave walker of this path can lead those individuals to new and exciting lives with higher levels of attainment on Maslow's hierarchy.

As Abraham Maslow said, "What is necessary to change a person is to change his awareness of himself."

Or when thinking about whether it makes sense to do, based on the *common sense* of society. What would Albert Einstein say about common sense. "Common sense is the collection of prejudices acquired by age eighteen." Our paradigms and beliefs about what a man is, what's right, and what's wrong, what's *normal* and what isn't, and a host of societal beliefs are stuck in our heads by the age of eighteen to rarely be reviewed and questioned. Maybe this is worth exploring to gain further growth as a person. You decide if you have the courage to grow through this, or the courage to help other's grow.

In any case, exploration and growth cannot happen when one does nothing. Go ahead. Stick that toe into that icy water and see if you too can warm it up and turn it into a spa, individually or together. Should you or the person you know chose to, or not, we wish you good luck and happy travels on the journey of growth and attainment!

If you enjoyed this book, it would be great if you could leave a review telling everyone how it was for you. Tell a friend about it. Blog it out. Any help is greatly appreciated. Thanks!

Barb and Thom

For more of our books, both fiction and non-fiction, go to:

Amazon:

http://www.amazon.com/Barbara-Deloto/e/B00J21HWA4/

Don't forget our website, which has more links to things you might like, as well as other places to get our works.

http://www.ShapeShifterBook.com

Barbara Deloto and Thomas Newgen

23

www.ingramcontent.com/pod-product-compliance
Lightning Source LLC
Chambersburg PA
CBHW031915270726
48655CB00003BA/1309